Top Essential Oil Recipes

BY LINDSEY P

A Recipe Guide Of Natural, Non-Toxic Aromatherapy & Essential Oils for Healing Common Ailments, Beauty, Stress & Anxiety

Table of Contents

Introduction

I want to thank you and congratulate you for downloading the book, *"Top Essential Oil Recipes: A Recipe Guide Of Natural, Non-Toxic Aromatherapy & Essential Oils for Healing common ailments, beauty, Stress & Anxiety."*

This book contains proven steps and strategies on how to use and combine essential oils to help alleviate anxiety issues and address health and beauty concerns. You will also be introduced to the basics of essential oils, how they are produced, and how they must be used.

Thanks again for purchasing this book, I hope you enjoy it!

Chapter 1: What Are Essential Oils?

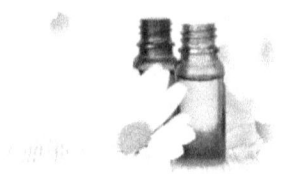

Have you ever squeezed a ripe orange peel? Surely you have noticed the fragrant residue on your hand? That residue is one example of an essential oil. Essential oils are naturally fragrant, highly concentrated compounds that can be obtained from myriad flowers, bark, roots, leaves, stems, seeds, and other plant parts. Each type of essential oil has their own characteristic scent that a person can immediately identify with one whiff.

Essential oils are fat soluble but they are not "oily" at all. They do not contain any fatty acids or lipids that are present in animal and vegetable oils. They also evaporate into the air unlike other oils. Essential oils are pure and very clean in a sense. When touched, it is immediately absorbed by the skin. Essential oils vary in colors. Untainted oils are usually translucent but some oils can be amber to deep blue in color.

Healing Effects of Essential Oils

Even though you might have heard of them recently, essential oils have actually been used for thousands of years. The ancient people rely on essential oils to heal and purify the body of ailments and diseases. When science and technology had taken over, the usage of these oils had greatly diminished since individuals have come to rely on drugs. But because of the myriad side effects of drugs, people are now opting for natural remedies including the use of essential oils. Apart from it medicinal properties, these powerful oils are also used for their cosmetic properties and emotionally uplifting benefits.

How to Use Essential Oils

Essential oils are not supposed to be applied directly on the skin unless appropriately diluted. This is because the potency of these oils can cause an allergic reaction on people with very sensitive skin. Here are some of the most common ways to use essential oils:

- Humidifier The essential oil's scent always calms and rejuvenates the senses. Alleviate symptoms of breathing in very dry air by adding a few drops of your favorite oil to a room humidifier. Not only will you breathe in scented, moist air but your asthma, sinusitis, and other related ailments will be put to a stop.

- Inhalation – If you don't have a humidifier, you can add a few drops of the essential oil into a small bowl of hot water. Put a towel over your head and inhale the aromatic steam vapors. If you have some trouble sleeping, you can strategically place a drop or two of the oil on your pillow to help relax yourself. If you are out of the home frequently, invest in a blank personal inhaler. This will allow you carry essential oil blends to rejuvenate or calm you anytime, anywhere.

- Bath Soak – Soaking in warm bathwater mixed with a few drops of essential oil helps remove stress, body pains, and heal minor skin diseases.

- Compress – Add about 5 drops (or more if you prefer) of essential oil to a small bowl of hot water. Soak a washcloth and wring out any excess. Place the towel on the part of your body that needs relief.

- Massage oil – Mixing a few drops of essential oil to a tablespoon of sweet almond oil, coconut oil, or grapeseed oil makes a perfect massage oil to soothe any bodily aches and pains.

- Diffuse – Instead of using a chemical-based air freshener, use essential oils instead. Place your oil inside a diffuser to dispense them into the hair. Not only will your home smell nice but you'll be relaxed as well.

- Dryer Sheet – Stop buying scented dryer sheets and make your own. Just add a few drops of your favorite oil fragrance to a piece of clean cloth and put in the dryer together with your clothes.

Chapter 2: Essential Oil Basics

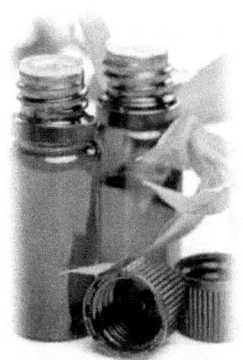

Now that you are showing an interest in essential oils, it is best that you, at least, know the basic things about them.

- It is very important to note that essential oils, although equally aromatic, are not the same with perfume and fragrance oils. Perfume and fragrance oils are created artificially, may contain chemicals, and don't have any therapeutic properties.

- Essential oils do not accumulate in the body. Once their healing properties are absorbed, they will be excreted naturally.

- Apart from water, essential oils can be diluted in carrier oils. Carrier oils are often unscented but others may have a faintly nutty or sweet fragrance. Perfect carrier oils for essential oils include sweet almond oil, pomegranate seed oil, evening primrose oil, olive oil, sesame oil, sunflower oil, hemp seed oil, jojoba, avocado oil, pecan oil, rose hip oil, and many more.

- Before using an essential oil for the first time, combine a drop of it to half a teaspoon of jojoba or olive oil. Rub the mixture on the inside of your wrist or upper arm. If there's no itching or redness after a few hours, the essential oil is safe for you to use. Remember, there's a great chance that you are allergic to essential oils if you have food allergies.

- Although most essential oils should never be used undiluted, small amounts of oils like lavender, tea tree, rose geranium, sandalwood, and German chamomile can be applied directly on the skin if used sparingly.

- Nursing women should steer clear from any type of essential oils. Pregnant women can use select oils sparingly only after the first trimester and upon the approval of a doctor.

- Never put essential oil on a baby or child's skin unless undiluted and half of the amount than a recipe calls for. Children have delicate, thin skin that may be damaged by the oil's potency. Essential oils that are safe for baby's include:

  a. Ginger

  b. Lemon

  c. Cypress

  d. Rosewood

  e. Rosemary

  f. Bergamot

  g. Roman Chamomile

  h. Lavender

  i. Orange

  j. Rose Otto

  k. Cedarwood

  l. Marjoram

  m. Mandarin

  n. Thyme

o. Ylang-Ylang

p. Melaleuca-Tea Tree

q. Frankincense

r. Geranium

s. Sandalwood

- Essential oils can be tested of its purity. Pour a single drop on a piece of clean construction paper. It should evaporate quickly without any traces. If there's a noticeable ring, it means that the oil is diluted.

- Pure essential oils can last you 5 to 10 years depending on your usage. These oils are so potent that you'll only need a couple of drops for each use. Most oils stay potent even after a decade except for citrus oils, which may deteriorate after two years.

- Store all your essential oil in a dark glass container/bottle in a cool and dark place that's away from direct sunlight. This will help preserve their volume and potency.

- No matter how delicious these essential oils smell, you should never ingest it. These oils are meant to be used externally and not for consumption. If you have small children in the home, it is best to keep it away of their reach.

Chapter 3: Making Essential Oils

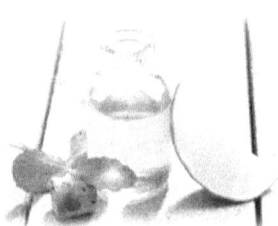

To make essential oils, it needs to be extracted from the plant. This can be done through expression and distillation.

Expression

Also referred as cold pressing, expression is method used to extract oils from citrus fruits like lime, orange, tangerine, lemon, and bergamot. In the past, expression doesn't require any sorts of tools except for a sponge. After soaking the citrus rind or zest, it will be pressed against the sponge repeatedly to absorb the oil. The sponge will then be squeezed over a container to catch the oils and allow it to separate from its juices. After a few hours, the oils will be siphoned off and bottled.

A modern type of expression involves using a blender-like device that's equipped with spikes. Once the citrus zest, rind, or peel is placed into the device, it will rotate and prod and prick the citrus until the oils are released. Oil will be collected at the bottom of the device and bottled immediately.

Distillation

Most essential oils are extracted using the distillation process. In this process, the plant part is placed on a grid that's inside a container called still. The still is then sealed. The water, steam, or water/steam combination swirling inside the sealed still will slowly break down the plant to release its volatile components and turn it into steam. These components will then rise up and collect into the condenser. Once the condenser is cool, the components will revert back into liquid form and will be collected in a separate container.

Once the essential oil separates from the water, it will be siphoned off and stored.

Extraction

Essential oils can also be extracted by using alcohol. The dried plant material is usually soaked in vodka or undenatured ethyl alcohol for several day until a substantial amount of oil is produced.

DIY or Purchase?

When it comes to essential oils, is it advantageous to make your own or buy from a trusted supplier?

Purchasing essential oils can get really expensive especially if you will be buying several oils all at once. Although each bottle of essential oil will last a long time, the amount that you pay upon the initial purchase can sting. The advantage of buying essential oils from a reputable brand is that you can be sure of its potency and quality.

Making your own essential oils is possible most especially if you have the time, patience, tools, and ingredients needed. If you already have everything you need, the cost of making your own essential oil will be minuscule. However, it is very important to note that DIY extraction of essential oils can lower its quality and potency unless you really are a pro. You would also need thousands of pounds of plant materials just to create a pound of a particular oil. You also need to make sure that it is very clean and free of chemicals like pesticides, herbicides, and the like.

All in all, it is best if you buy essential oils than make it yourself. Aside from being hassle-free, you can buy small quantities of several oils all at once. The more essential oils you have, the more chances you have of experiencing its benefits.'

Mixing and Matching Essential Oils

Now that you own several essential oils, you'll be glad to know that you can easily combine to create a concoction that can heal, relax, and beautify you. This powerful mixture is called a synergy blend. Synergy blend oils are combinations of different oils with complementing properties. These oil blends can be utilized for either aromatherapy, medicinal, or cosmetic purposes.

Chapter 4: Essential Oil Recipes for Various Ailments

Pain

If you are in pain, concoct one of these essential oil recipes to get relief. Place all the needed oils in a small bottle, cap tightly, and shake well to mix. Then, massage on the affected areas (unless stated otherwise) whenever needed.

Nerve Pain

4 drops chamomile oil

3 drops helichrysum oil

3 drops marjoram oil

2 drops lavender oil

1 ounce St. John's wort oil

Stomach Pain

1 drop chamomile oil

1 drop peppermint oil

1 drop clove oil

2 drops rosemary oil

5ml vegetable carrier oil

Headaches

10 drops of peppermint oil

8 drops marjoram oil

10 drops basil oil

3 drops helichrysm oil

Injury

10 drops lavender oil

10 drops cypress oil

15 drops deep blue oil

10 drops sandalwood oil

20 drops marjoram oil

20 drops lemon grass oil

10ml vegetable carrier oil

Pulled Muscle

2 drops sweet marjoram oil

3 drops Roman chamomile oil

*apply via cold compress

Muscle Pain

a. Blend 1

3 drops lavender oil

3 drops Roman chamomile oil

*apply via cold compress

b. Blend 2

5 drops rosemary oil

10 drops lavender oil

15 drops cypress oil

½ ounce sunflower oil

Tight Muscles

4 drops rosemary oil

4 drops lavender oil

2 drops ginger oil

4 teaspoons sweet almond oil

Sore Muscles

a. Blend 1

5 drops peppermint oil

10 drops rosemary oil

5 drops Roman chamomile oil

5 drops lavender oil

5 drops lemon oil

1 ounce sweet almond oil

b. Blend 2

20 drops Ylang-Ylang oil

12 drops nutmeg oil

20 drops ginger oil

8 drops rosemary oil

2   ounces sweet almond oil

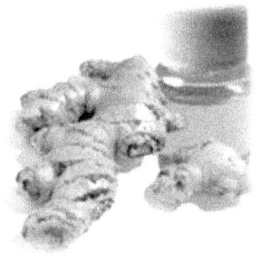

Blend 3

4 drops rosemary oil

4 drops bay laurel oil

3 drops Ylang-Ylang oil

4 drops eucalyptus oil

15ml carrier oil

Rheumatic Pain

4 drops ginger oil

2 drops spike lavender oil

4 drops silver fir oil

4 teaspoons carrier oil

Leg Cramps

2 drops ginger oil

4 drops cinnamon oil

4 drops black pepper oil

4 teaspoons carrier oil

Back Pains

a. Blend 1

10 drops lavender oil

6 drops sandalwood oil

6 drops rosemary oil

3 drops geranium oil

2 tablespoons almond oil

b. Blend 2

4 drops cardamom oil

4 drops ginger oil

4 drops wintergreen

15ml sweet almond oil

For Assorted Health Concerns

Eczema Cream

25 drops Melrose oil

25 drops lavender oil

½ cup coconut oil (solid)

Put all the ingredients in a mixing bowl. Using a stand mixer, whip at medium-high speed until thick and peaky. Store the cream in small, wide-mouth glass jars. Apply on the skin before sleeping until skin condition improves.

Cough Blend

1 drop peppermint oil

1 drop pine needle oil

1 drop eucalyptus globulus

Put the oils in a small bowl of steaming hot water. Inhale the steam to loosen mucus and get relief.

Cold Relief

2 drops rosemary oil

2 drops peppermint oil

2 drops eucalyptus globulus oil

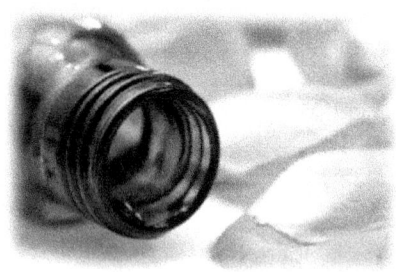

Blend the oils together in a bottle and add a few drops in your personal inhaler. Place the inhaler near your nostrils and inhale slowly to get relief.

Fever Reducer

For kids 3 months to 6 years old:

5 drops chamomile oil

3 drops lavender oil

2 drops frankincense oil

For kids 6 to 10 years old:

2 drops frankincense

3 drops peppermint oil

5 drops rosemary oil

To use, place the selected oil blend in a steam vaporizer or oil diffuser. You can also dilute the oils with 1 ounce of carrier oil and apply it to the child's body.

Bruise Be Gone

8 drops helichrysum oil

1 ounce sweet almond oil

Put the oils in a bottle and shake well to combine. Apply lightly on the bruises several times a day.

Athlete's Foot Fighter

3 drops thyme oil

8 drops geranium oil

12 drops tea tree oil

2 drops myrrh (optional)

2 ounces apple cider vinegar

1 tablespoon tincture of benzoin

Mix all the ingredients together and apply on the affected area. Apply several times a day.

Tooth Pain Relief

1 teaspoon vegetable oil

1 drop orange oil

4 drops clove bud oil

Combine the ingredients together. Rub on the gums every half hour or as needed. This recipe may also be used on children.

Sore Throat Gargle

½ cup warm water

4 drop marjoram oil

½ teaspoon sea salt

Combine all the ingredients in a cup. Stir well to dissolve the salt and break up oil. Gargle every 30 minutes each day to get relief.

Herpes Relief

5 drops bergamot oil

5 drops myrrh oil

10 drops tea tree oil

2 drops peppermint oil (optional)

½ ounce vegetable oil

Combine all the ingredients and stir well. The addition of the peppermint oil in the recipe is optional as some people find that it increases the pain. If you can tolerate it, the better. Apply directly on the affected area several times a day.

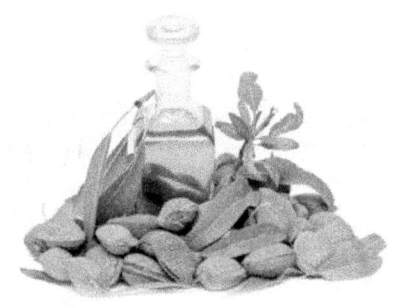

Dermatitis Balm

8 drops chamomile oil

8 drops tea tree oil

2 ounces healing balm

1 teaspoon Oregon grape tincture

Use a toothpick to stir the oils and tincture into the healing balm. Once mixed, apply the balm 3 to 4 times a day to the afflicted area of the skin.

Inhalation Rub for Asthma

6 drops lavender oil

1 drop marjoram oil

4 drops geranium oil

1 drop ginger oil

1 ounce vegetable oil

Mix all the ingredients in a small bowl. Rub on the asthmatic's chest before bedtime and instruct him to inhale a few times before lying down. Repeat for several nights.

Bladder Infection Reliever

2 drops fennel oil

8 drops cypress oil

6 drops bergamot oil

6 drops tea tree oil

2 ounces vegetable oil

Mix all the ingredients and massage over your lower abdomen. You may also add a few drops of the oil blend to your warm bath.

Cold and Flu energizer

10 drops eucalyptus oil

4 drops peppermint oil

10 drops ravensara oil

8 drops rosemary oil

Blend the ingredients together in a bowl. Pour into your bath water. This is a stimulating blend which can help relive cold and flu symptoms.

Menstrual cramps relief

1 oz jojoba oil

4 drops cypress essential oil

4 drops peppermint oil

3 drops lavender essential oil

Menstrual cramps can be very uncomfortable and can also hinder you from enjoying other activities. Simply mix the oils together and store in a dark bottle until ready to use. Pour a small amount into your palms and massage in your abdomen.

Anti-inflammation blend

8 drops roman chamomile

3 drops lime oil

1 oz jojoba oil

Mix the lime and roman chamomile oil then add to the jojoba oil. Store in a glass container then apply to inflamed areas around your body.

Citronella Insect Repellant

10 drops lavender essential oil

5 drops lemongrass essential oil

15 drops essential oil

10 drops eucalyptus essential oil

1.5 oz distilled water

Pour the distilled water into the bottle. Gently add the oils then shake the bottle before using. Remember that oil and water do not mix well together so it is normal if you see the oil float on top. Mist into your skin or clothes as needed.

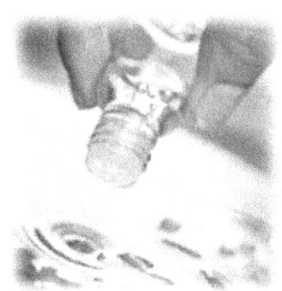

Intensive Nausea relief

2 drops lemongrass oil

2 drops chamomile oil

1 drop fennel oil

2 oz vegetable oil

Mix the ingredients and use it to massage in your abdominal area. This blend can help with indigestion, gas and motion sickness. You can also add it to your bath water.

Eye strain therapy

2 bags of chamomile tea

1 drop of chamomile oil

1 drop of lavender oil

Eye strain is common for people with desk jobs that involve computers. Seep the tea bags in hot water. Allow to cool enough then add the essential oil. Be careful not to add too much. Lie down and place the bags over your closed eyes.

Ear ache remedy

3 drops tea tree oil

1 tbsp vegetable oil

3 drops lavender oil

Earaches are often caused by infection. Combine the ingredients in a bowl then rub the oil on the side of your neck. Use only half of the recipe if you plan to use it on children.

Chest congestion relief diffuser

5 drops eucalyptus oil

3 drops rose oil

¼ tsp coarse salt

Place the salt in a small glass bottle then add the oil. The salt will absorb the oil. Inhale from the bottle. You can carry the mixture in your bag and sniff throughout the day as needed.

Instant relief vapor rub

5 drops peppermint oil

10 drops eucalyptus oil

1 oz coconut oil

5 drops chamomile oil

The common cause of lung congestion is cold and flu virus. Mix the ingredients in a bottle then shake well to combine. Massage the oil into your chest and throat area. You can use this blend five times in a day.

Immunity boosting tonic blend

6 drops lavender oil

3 drops citrus oil

2 drops myrrh oil

6 drops bergamot oil

3 drops tea tree oil

2 oz coconut oil

Combine all of the ingredients then use as massage oil all over your body. You can also add it to your bath water. Use several times a day to improve your natural immunity.

Lavender compress for varicose veins

3 drops chamomile oil

 3 drops lavender oil

1 tsp St. John wort

3 drops carrot seed oil

1 cup cold water

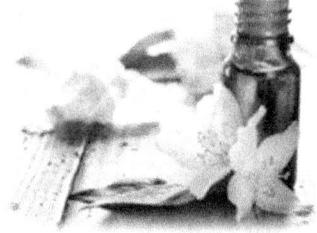

Combine the ingredients then pour into a soft cloth. Wring it then place over your various veins. It can be used daily. This blend can also be used to treat hemorrhoids.

Easy headache cure compress

5 drops lavender/ eucalyptus oil

1 cup cold water

Add the oil into the water. Use a soft cloth and submerge it into the mixture. Place the cloth over your eyes and forehead.

Migraine relief blend

1 quart hot water

5 drops lavender oil

5 drops ginger oil

Gently add the oil into the hot water then soak your feet into the mixture for several minutes.

Hives skin wash

5 drops chamomile oil

3 tbsp baking soda

3 drops peppermint oil

2 cups water

Hives are rashes-like bumps that appear on the skin surface. It is often caused by food allergy. Mix the ingredients in a large bowl. You can alternatively use tea water instead of plain water. Pour into a damp cloth then apply to the skin to relive itching.

Germ fighting blend for cuts

2 oz distilled water

6 drops eucalyptus oil

12 drops tea tree oil

6 drops lemon oil

Mix the ingredients and shake well to combine. Pour the mixture into a spray bottle then apply on minor cuts and burns. You can also apply antiseptic herb like Oregon grape root.

Acne treatment

Acne prone skin needs special care. Adding natural treatment to your regime can help reduce and even eliminate acne.

- Acne spot treatment

2 drops manuka essential oil

2 drops castor seed oil

1 oz jojoba oil

3 drops camphor oil

4 drops sweet orange oil

Combine the ingredient in a glass bottle. To use, spread a single drop of the mixture to the affected area for best results.

- Anti-acne cream

4 tsp grape seed oil

½ tsp stearic acid

½ tsp vitamin E

1 tbsp aloe vera gel

5 drops lavender oil

1 drop ylang ylang

1 drop cedar wood oil

1 tbsp emulsifying wax

1/3 cup water or witch hazel

5 drops grape fruit extract

3 drops lemon essential oil

Stir the oil, wax and acid in a measuring cup. Place it over warm water then simmer. Stir occasionally until the wax is melted. Add the vitamin E. Pour the witch hazel and aloe vera in the cup. Microwave it for few seconds. Combine the oils and witch hazel mixture. Stir constantly then pour the mixture in a clean jar. Stir the cream occasionally to prevent the ingredients from separating.

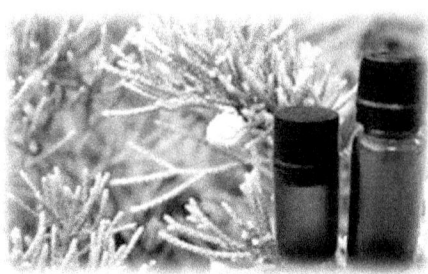

Chapter 5: Essential Oils Recipes for Stress and Anxiety

Mood Enhancer Natural Parfum

1 teaspoon fractionated coconut oil (melted)

1 drop bergamot oil

1 drop Ylang-Ylang oil

3 drops clary sage

4 drops tangerine oil

3 drops lavender oil

Put all the oils inside a roller bottle. Shake well before using.

Depression Lifter Spray

3 drops petitgrain Oil

6 drops bergamot oil

1 drop neroli oil (can be optional)

3 drops geranium oil

2 ounces water

Put all ingredients inside a spray bottle and shake well to blend. Spritz over your face or body whenever needed.

Anger Away Blend

4 drops Ylang-Ylang oil

3 drops cypress oil

2 drops frankincense oil

4 drops patchouli oil

2 drops clary sage

7 drops geranium

5 drops bergamot

Put all the ingredients inside a small bottle. Close and shake well. Rub small amounts of the oil over the heart and liver areas as well as on the bottoms of the feet.

For Emotional Release

15 drops sandalwood oil

25 drops geranium oil

30 drops Ylang-Ylang oil

10 drops ledum oil

20 drops German chamomile oil

Put all the oils in a bottle. Secure cap and shake well. Rub a small amount on your chest and back.

Pick Me Upper

5 drops spearmint oil

10 drops bergamot oil

10 drops grapefruit oil

Put all the oils in a bottle and mix well. Add several drops in a diffuser to lighten your mood.

Ease the Panic Blend

1 drop rose oil

20 drops bergamot oil

15 drops lavender oil

5 drops basil oil

3 drops neroli oil

Mix all the oils in a glass bottle by shaking vigorously. Put several drops in your personal inhaler whenever you feel panic settling in. You may also use a diffuser.

Slow Down Blend

1 drop lavender oil

1 drop Ylang-Ylang oil

1 drop bergamot oil

1 drop patchouli oil

Combine all the oils in a small bottle and shake well. Add a few drops in a diffuser to relax.

Comforting Body Spray

15 drops sweet orange oil

10 drops cinnamon leaf oil

8 ounces distilled water

1 tablespoon witch hazel

a spray bottle

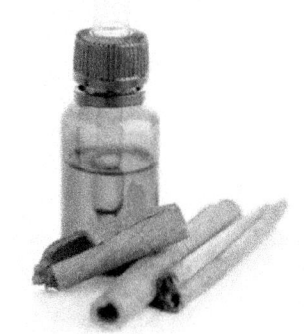

Pour all the ingredients inside the spray bottle. Close and shake well. Spray on your body whenever needed. Store in the fridge and use within two weeks.

Perk My Energy Blend

2 drops eucalyptus oil

2 drops peppermint oil

8 drops lemon oil

1 drop cinnamon leaf oil

1 drop cardamom oil

2 ounces vegetable oil

Combine all the ingredients and use to massage the entire body. Use as often as needed.

Memory Enhancer

1 drop clary sage oil

6 drops lemon oil

10 drops rosemary oil

Combine all the oils in a bottle and shake well. Add a few drops to your personal inhaler and smell while studying. You may also use the oil in your diffuser.

Sleep Inducer

10 drops sandalwood

10 drops lavender oil

15 drops bergamot oil

2 drops Ylang-Ylang oil

3 drops frankincense oil

4 ounces vegetable oil

Mix all the ingredients together and massage all over the body. You can also add 2 teaspoons to your warm bath.

Stress remedy inhaler

10 drops bergamot essential oil

4 drops orange essential oil

1 drop ylang ylang oil

4 drops lavender oil

1 drop rose geranium oil

1 tsp salt

Combine the ingredients together in a dark bottle. To use, take three long whiffs from the bottle and take a rest before repeating the process.

Mandarin and lavender bath salts

12 drops mandarin oil

8 drops lavender oil

1 cup Epsom bath salt

Combine the ingredients and store in a glass container. Add to your water before bathing.

Super-relaxing bath oil

30 drops sandalwood oil

2 drops cedar wood oil

125 ml carrier oil such as sweet almond oil or jojoba oil

12 drops lavender oil

Mix all of the ingredients in a dark glass bottle. Store it in a dark and cool place. Pour a tablespoon of the mixture in your bath water.

Chapter 6: Essential Oil Blends for Cosmetic Use

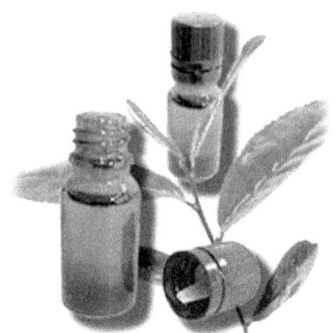

Make your own natural beauty products by using essential oils as ingredients. Try these recipes:

Peppermint Rosemary Shampoo

2 drops peppermint oil

16 drops rosemary oil

½ cup distilled water

½ cup castile soap

Obtain a clean flip top container and put in the castile soap. Add the peppermint and rosemary oil before adding the water. Close the container and shake before using.

Oily Skin Toner

1 drop rose geranium oil

3 drops palmarosa oil

3 drops lemongrass oil

3 drops petitgrain oil

3 drops tea tree oil

1 cup witch hazel

Mix all the ingredients and apply on the face using a cotton ball. Let dry.

Honey Lavender Lip Balm

15 drops lavender oil

5 drops Frankincense oil

1 tablespoon sweet almond oil

½ teaspoon raw honey

2 tablespoon coconut oil

2 tablespoon beeswax

1 tablespoon raw honey

1 rubber band (large)

12 lip balm tubes

Remove the caps from all tubes and position them upright using the rubber band. Using a double broiler, melt the honey, coconut oil, shea butter, and beeswax. Remove from heat once melted and mix in the essential oils and sweet almond oil. Carefully pour the mixture into the tubes, dividing them equally. Let the balm set before recapping the tubes.

Extra Strength Blemish Mask

800 units Vitamin E

12 drops tea tree oil

½ teaspoon Oregon grape root powder

Several drops of water

Stir the oil into the powder. Add water by drop until a paste is formed. Apply the mask on the entire face and let dry. Wait for 20 minutes before rinsing.

Shaving Cream

12 drops pure lavender oil

2 tablespoons sweet almond oil

3 tablespoons coconut oil

4 tablespoon shea butter (solid)

Use a double broiler to melt the coconut oil and shea butter over a low heat. Stir until completely melted. Add the remaining oils and mix well. Put in the fridge and let harden for a few hours. Remove from the fridge and whip until a frosting-like consistency is achieved. Let it sit for a few minutes before transferring to an airtight jar.

Lemon Honey Body Scrub

¼ cup olive oil

15 drops lavender oil

15 drops lemon oil

2 teaspoons dried rosemary

2 tablespoons raw honey

1 cup organic cane sugar

Mix the rosemary, raw honey, and sugar with the olive oil. Add in the essential oils and stir thoroughly. Use immediately or you can store it in a glass container for later use. This scrub lasts up to 2 to 3 months.

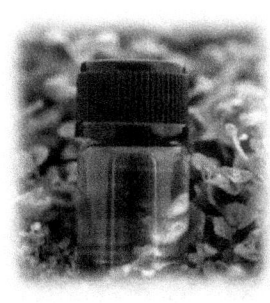

Homemade EO Toothpaste

20 drops peppermint oil

10 drops trace minerals

2 tablespoons coconut oil

2 tablespoons calcium magnesium powder

2 tablespoons baking soda

2 tablespoons real sea salt

2 tablespoons xylitol powder

Mix all powdered ingredients first. Add the coconut oil one tablespoon at a time. Add the salt and the peppermint oil. Mix thoroughly and store in a jar with a secure lid.

Solid Perfumes

- **Deep and Sensual Scent**

  10 drops sandalwood oil

  20 drops sweet orange oil

  15 drops Ylang-Ylang oil

- **Fresh and Spicy Scent**

  10 drops vetiver oil

17 drops grapefruit oil

14 drops ginger oil

- **Romantic and Whimsical Scent**

10 drops vetiver oil

25 drops rose oil

10 drops lime oil

Choose the scent of your choice and prepare the essential oils needed. Use double broiler and melt 2 teaspoon grated beeswax. Turn off the heat and add in 2 teaspoon sweet almond oil. Mix well and add the appropriate essential oils. Pour the mixture into your desired container and let harden. To use: rub a finger into the solid perfume before wiping it on your skin.

Soothing Natural Deodorant

3 tablespoons apricot kernel oil

5 tablespoons coconut oil

2 tablespoons dried calendula

3 tablespoons dried chamomile

10 drops tea tree oil

10 drops lavender oil

¼ cup + 2 tablespoons arrow root powder

¼ cup + 2 tablespoons baking soda

Liquefy the coconut oil using a double broiler or the microwave. Put it in a sterilized jar and add in the apricot kernel oil. Put in the dried calendula and dried chamomile in the jar and seal tightly. Shake well until the flowers are completely soaked. Store in a dark place for 3 weeks, shaking the jar daily.

After the appropriate time, strain the infused oil and remove the flowers. You may need to heat up the oil if it has solidified. In another jar, mix the infused oil, the arrow root powder, and baking soda. Mix well. Add the essential oils per drop while stirring. Use within 3 months.

Hair Styling Wax

10 drops rosemary oil

10 drops peppermint oil

0.75 ounce beeswax

0.75 ounce fractionated coconut oil

0.5 ounce shea butter

Put the beeswax, coconut oil, and shea butter in a double broiler. Stir until completely melted. Turn off the heat and let cool for about 3 minutes. Add the oils and mix well. Transfer the mixture into a lidded glass jar. Let rest for two hours before using. Using your fingers, apply a small amount on the hair and style as usual.

Natural Sunscreen

1 teaspoon vitamin E

2 tablespoons zinc oxide

12 drops helichrysum oil

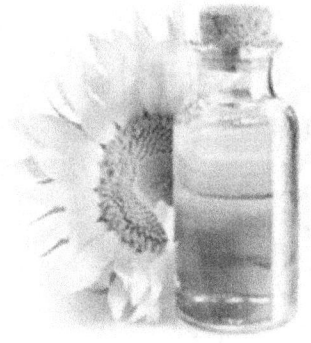

2 tablespoons shea butter

¼ cup beeswax

¼ cup fractionated coconut oil

¼ cup olive oil

Place the vitamin E, shea butter, beeswax, coconut oil, and olive oil in a double broiler. Over medium heat, stir the ingredients until thoroughly melted. Remove from heat and let cool. Add the helichrysum oil and the zinc oxide to the mix. Combine well. Store in a jar with lid and put in the refrigerator. This sunscreen must be used within 6 months of creation.

Talc-Free Powder

½ cup arrowroot powder

½ cup cornstarch

½ cup oats (finely ground)

2 drops lavender oil

1 drop Roman chamomile oil

Mix all the ingredients well and store in a shaker bottle.

Moisturizing Facial Oil

Base oils:

Argan oil (for aging, dry, oily, and acne-prone skin)

Jojoba oil (for aging, dry, oily, and acne-prone skin)

Grapeseed oil (for normal, oil, and acne-prone skin)

Nourishing oils:

> Sea buckthorn oil – nourishing and perfect for all skin types

> Rosehip seed oil – regenerating, firming, and perfect for all skin types especially aging skin

> Borage oil – perfect for oily and acne-prone skin

> Evening primrose skin – perfect for all skin types

Essential Oils:

> Lavender – a healing oil that's perfect for all skin types

> Peppermint – astringent oil that's perfect for oily and acne-prone skin

> Rose – components are suitable for dry, aging, and normal skin.

> Rosemary – for acne-prone and oily skin

Choose one of each base oil, nourishing oil, and essential oil that's suitable for your skin type. Fill a 1-ounce bottle and fill the bottle almost halfway with your base oil. Add in your nourishing oil. The bottle should be almost full at this time. Lastly, add 5 to 7 drops of the essential oil of your choice. If using peppermint, you might want to add only about 3 to 4 drops. Shake well. Store away from direct sunlight and use within one year.

Dry Shampoo

2 drops peppermint oil

2 drops rosemary oil

2 drops lavender oil

*¼ cup arrowroot powder

*for dark hair, use 2 tablespoons arrowroot powder and 2 tablespoons of cocoa powder

Combine all ingredients in a food processor. Pulse until thoroughly blended. Store in a wide mouth jar. Apply the powder to the roots of the hair using an old makeup brush.

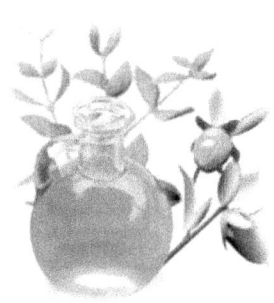

Nail and Cuticle Care

3 drops lemon oil

3 drops geranium oil

3 drops rosemary oil

6 drops clary sage

6 drops lavender

1 ounce sweet almond oil

1 ounce jojoba

Put all the oil inside a bottle and shake to blend well. At bedtime, put a drop on each of your fingernail and massage. This will help soften the cuticles and harden the nails.

Anti-Itch Lotion

10 drops German chamomile

20 drops lavender

5 drops peppermint

10 eucalyptus globulus

Mix all the oils together and add to **2 ounces of lotion** (unscented). Stir well. Apply to itchy area to get relief.

Basic Organic Lotion

½ cup olive oil

¼ cup beeswax

2 tbsp cocoa butter

¼ cup coconut oil

10 drops rose oil

10 drops cinnamon oil

Combine the ingredients in a large jar. Pour water in a medium pan then place it over medium heat. Secure the lid of the jar and place into the pan. As the water begins to boil, the contents of the jar will also start to melt. Stir occasionally. Set aside and allow it to cool. Use it like a regular lotion.

Nourishing essential oil lotion

10 drops patchouli

5 drops carrot seed

25 drops sandalwood

8 oz unscented body oil

Pour the lotion in a mixing bowl then add the essential oils. Mix together to combine then pour back into the container.

Calming lavender lotion

1/3 cup coconut oil

5 drops lavender oil

2 tbsp beeswax

Place all of the ingredients in a pan and place it over medium heat. Wait until it is fully melted. Use an electric mixer to whip the lotion. Pour the mixture into a glass container and seal.

Herb-infused hair detangling spray

1.5 cups distilled water

2 tbsp conditioner of choice

3 tbsp marshmallow root

10 drops rose oil

5 drops chamomile oil

Boil the water in the pan. Allow to simmer for 30 minutes. Allow the mixture to cool slightly and strain the mixture over a thin cloth. Pour in the bottle then add the conditioner and essential oils. Shake until it is well combined. This can be stored for up to two months.

Lime hand sanitizer

2 tsp aloe vera gel

10 drops vitamin E oil

10 drops lime oil

10 drops lavender oil

10 drops melaleuca oil

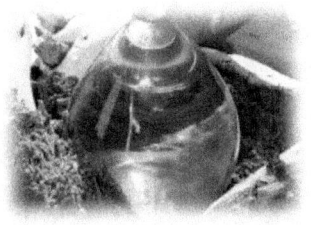

Use a glass pray bottle for this hand sanitizer. Fill it with half of the water. Add the vitamin E, aloe vera gel and oils. Add the remaining water then shake to combine. Simply spray into hands and rub together.

Vanilla sugar scrub

½ cup brown sugar

1/3 cup coconut oil

¼ tsp pure vanilla extract

½ tsp vitamin E oil

½ cup granulated sugar

10 drops chamomile oil

Combine the ingredients together in a small container. To use, simply apply to your skin. Be careful not to rub too vigorously and avoid the eye area completely. Wash with warm water then finish it off with cold water.

Peppermint body butter

½ cup coconut oil

½ cup shea butter

1 tsp vitamin E oil

4 drops peppermint oil

½ cup sweet almond oil

½ cup cocoa butter

Place the shea butter, coconut oil and cocoa butter in a pot then place it over low heat. Combine the ingredients together until it is fully melted. Remove it from the heat. Mix in the vitamin E, peppermint oil and sweet almond oil. Place in the refrigerator for an hour. Once chilled, use a hand mixer to stir the body butter. Transfer the mixture in a glass jar.

Relaxing bath melts

50 grams shea butter

¼ tsp honey lavender organic tea

30 drops lavender oil

50 grams cocoa butter

1 tsp lavender flowers

Scoop the shea butter and cocoa butter in a double broiler. Heat until the butter is melted. Break the tea bag and add the contents in the butter mixture. Stir it to combine. Pour the mixture into a small mold. Chill it for 30 minutes or until it hardens.

Lotion bars

Hard lotion bars are like liquid lotion but they stay solid at room temperature. It gently melts as you apply it to your skin. Your natural body warmth can soften the bar and allow it to glide smoothly in your skin.

- **Orange Honey Lotion bars**

1 ½ tbsp raw honey

2 oz organic shea butter

1 tbsp olive oil

2 oz organic beeswax

2 oz organic coconut oil

6 drops of sweet orange oil

Melt the butter in a pan then add the coconut oil and shea butter. Stir until it becomes smooth. Reduce the heat then add the remaining ingredients. Line the muffin tins with liners. Pour the mixture into the mold then allow to harden for several hours.

- **Coconut oil lotion bars**

1 cup coconut oil

5 ginger oil

10 drops lavender oil

1 cup pure beeswax

Heat the coconut oil and beeswax in a pan and place it over medium heat. You can also break the wax into small pieces. Add the essential oils and stir to combine. Pour the mixture into bar molds then allow it to cool.

- **Sunscreen lotion bars**

½ cup shea butter

½ cup coconut oil

½ tsp vitamin E oil

5 tbsp beeswax

2 tbsp zinc oxide

¾ tsp lavender oil

Mix the coconut oil, beeswax and butter in a pot over a double broiler. Heat until the ingredients is melted together. Remove it from the heat and stir to mix the ingredients. Add the other ingredients. Pour into a mold and place in the refrigerator for an hour or until it is solid.

- **Bug repellant lotion bars**

¼ cup coconut oil

¼ cup grated beeswax

5 drops citronella oil

3 drops lemongrass oil

3 drops rosemary oil

3 drops lavender oil

¼ cup cocoa butter

Set a glass bowl over a pot of boiling water. Melt the coconut oil, beeswax and cocoa butter. Stir to mix. Remove from the heat then add the Vitamin E. Pour it in a mold. Allow to cool before storing it.

Cleansing facial wipes

2 cups distilled water

5 drops tea tree essential oil

2 drops aloe vera oil

1 tbsp melted coconut oil

5 drops grapefruit oil

Cut an old white shirt or towel. Pour the melted coconut oil in a glass container then gently add the essential oils. Add the water and stir again. Layer the strips of cloth in the container and allow it to absorb the solution. Store it at room temperature. Use it like a regular face wipe.

Chocolate mint lip balm

2 tbsp coconut oil

1 tbsp sweet almond oil

¼ tsp peppermint oil

2 tbsp beeswax

1 tbsp cocoa butter

Melt the coconut oil, sweet almond oil, beeswax and cocoa butter in a broiler. Remove it from the heat then add the essential oils. Pour the mixture into the tubes. Make sure to move quickly since the mixture can harden pretty fast. Allow the lip balms to harden before you set the caps.

Natural tinted lip balm

2 tbsp coconut oil

2 tsp grated cocoa butter

1 tsp Vitamin E

2 tsp Hibiscus powder

2 tbsp jojoba oil

1 tbsp grated beeswax

½ tsp grapefruit oil

Melt the coconut oil, wax and butter in a pan. Stir until the fully incorporated. Add the oil, vitamin E and herbal powder. Mix until combined. Quickly stir the mixture and pour into a glass container.

Peppermint citrus scrubs

1 cup granulated sugar

1/3 cup coconut oil

4 tbsp orange zest

10 drops peppermint oil

2 tbsp vegetable glycerin

10 drops wild orange essential oil

Combine the glycerin, zest, oil and sugar in a container. You may need to add more oil to get the desired consistency. Add the essential oil then stir. Store it in a glass container. To use, rub a small amount into your skin and rinse with water.

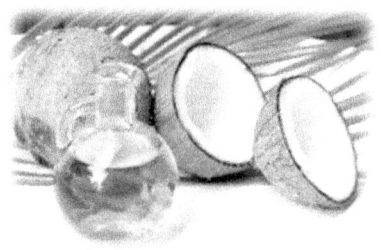

Natural mascara

2 tsp coconut oil

2 drops lavender oil

4 tsp aloe vera gel

2 capsules of activated charcoal for black mascara or cocoa powder for brown mascara

½ tsp beeswax

Pour the coconut oil, bees wax and aloe vera gel in a saucepan then simmer over low heat until the wax is melted.

Open and pour the activated charcoal into the mixture. Stir until well blended. Pour into a bag then cut one corner end. Use it like a piping bag to transfer the mascara mixture into an old clean mascara tube.

All natural foundation powder

Arrowroot powder

1 part ground cinnamon

1 part cocoa powder

1 part nutmeg

3 drops olive oil

3 drops almond oil

Start with the base powder. You can use 1 tsp for dark skin or 1 tbsp for lighter skin. Add the cocoa powder, nutmeg and cinnamon until you have your desired shade. Add the essential oils then stir to combine. Use a foundation brush to apply.

Bubble bath recipes

Bubble bath is a fun way to relax. You can experiment with different essential oils to see what works for you.

1 ½ cup liquid castile soap

½ tsp white sugar

2 tbsp vegetable glycerin

Choose one of the recipes below and create your own signature bubble bath.

- **Lavender lift**

4 drops lemon oil

1 drop chamomile oil

5 drops lavender oil

- **Smooth silk and spice**

5 drops lavender oil

1 drop patchouli oil

1 drop clove oil

- **Summer rose scent**

3 drops rose absolute oil

1 drop geranium oil

2 drops palmarosa oil

- **Sweet vanilla**

2 drops rose oil

10 drops vanilla oil

- **Sunny and citrus**

1 drop rose geranium oil

4 drops orange oil

5 drops bergamot oil

Gently add all of the ingredients together in a large glass container. Stir until the sugar is fully dissolved. Allow to sit for a day before using. To use, pour a handful into your bath water.

Natural hair dyes

Natural hair dyes may not be able to give you fast results like chemical based hair dyes but it can enhance your natural hair color and can create subtle highlight if used for a long time.

- ### Sage and rosemary dye for gray hair

2 cups hot water

½ cup dried rosemary leaves

½ cup dried sage leaves

4 drops lavender oil

Combine the ingredients in a pot then simmer over low heat for half an hour. Stain and use as a hair dye. Apply to your hair and leave it to dry. Rinse and dry. You will need to repeat this weekly until you obtain your desired shade. This mixture is safe to use every day.

- ### Hair dye for blonds

3 tbsp chamomile flowers

3 tbsp lemon peel

4 drops chamomile oil

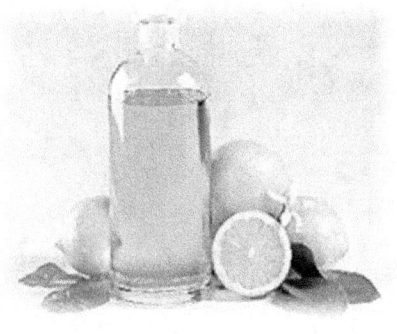

Combine the ingredients in a pot and simmer for several hours. Strain the liquid and transfer into a bottle. Add 2 tablespoon of apple cider vinegar. Pour in your hair and gently massage to the scalp. This mixture can also effectively remove shampoo buildup.

- **Marigold hair color for redheads**

1/3 cup marigold flowers

2 ½ cup distilled water

3 drops marigold oil

¼ cup red wine

Simmer the flowers then remove from the heat before adding the oil. Strain the liquid then add the red wine. Apply the liquid into your hair as a final rinse. Dry your hair in the sun if possible. This mixture adds subtle hints of red and gold highlights to your hair.

- **Rich brown hair dye for dark hair**

1/3 cup walnut shells

1/3 cup black tea

1/3 cup whole cloves

2 ½ cups distilled water

Combine the ingredients together in a pot. Remove from the heat and allow to cool. Strain the liquid and apply after shampooing. Use it every day until the desired color is achieved.

Hibiscus hair pack

3 oz hibiscus petal powder

6 tsp aloe vera gel

Coconut milk

10 drops peppermint oil

10 drops rosemary oil

3 tsp honey

3 tbsp plain yogurt

10 drops lemongrass essential oil

Combine the ingredients together in a bowl then add stir to make a paste. Massage into your hair and wrap it with plastic or you can use a shower cap. Leave the mixture in your hair for an hour. Rinse well. You can use this once a week.

Hair growth rinse

2 cups distilled water

3 tbsp dried rosemary

20 drops lavender oil

20 drops sage essential oil

3 tbsp dried sage

2 tbsp apple cider vinegar

20 drops rosemary oil

Combine the herbs and water in a pot then boil over medium heat. Allow to seep for three hours then strain the liquid. Pour into a bottle. Add the essential oil and vinegar. Stir to combine. Rub it in your hair and scalp. You can leave it to dry or rinse it with cold water.

Aloe vera scalp treatment

¼ cup aloe vera gel

12 drops lavender oil

3 drops cedar wood oil

10 drops rosemary oil

1 tsp jojoba oil

Mix the ingredients in a dark bottle. Massage the mixture into your scalp every night to increase blood flow and to stimulate hair follicles.

Chapter 7: Essential oil recipes for weight loss

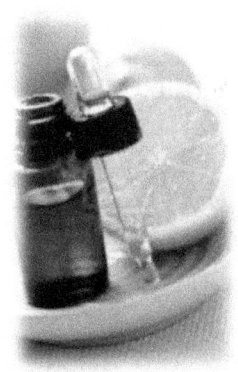

Using essential oils for weight loss can complement a healthy lifestyle change. It can help you get through a weight loss plateau or help you control your appetite. You can always find a holistic approach to address several health issues like your digestive health, metabolism, cravings and diet.

Top Essential Oils for Weight Loss

Grapefruit

Grapefruit oil is one of the top essential oils for weight loss. Grapefruit oil has been known to help prevent overeating. Others believe that grapefruit oil can reduce cellulite build-up in the body if it is applied as massage oil. It can also help tone the muscles. Studies also show that grapefruit extract can reduce fluid retention in the body and can even dissolve fat. People also notice that they feel slightly invigorated after smelling the oil.

Lemon

Lemon oil is a common ingredient in household cleaning products because of its antiseptic qualities. This oil can also gently detoxify the body and increase your energy levels. It can also address different digestive problems and can even help eliminate intestinal parasites.

Peppermint

This spicy and mint essential oil is great for digestive issues. It can also stimulate the mind and help you concentrate better. Studies show that it can help cure candida which often affects a person's weight. Peppermint oil can help you feel fuller for a longer time. Researchers suggest that it can affect a part of the brain that controls the feeling of satiety. Additionally, it can also increase motivation and optimism.

Ginger

Ginger is known to cure digestive problems. It can also effectively warm the body and increase your energy. Use it as a tonic to stimulate your system. Emotionally, ginger essential oil can increase sense of well being and helps to create empowerment. It can stimulate your inner strength and helps you cope with change.

Cinnamon

Cinnamon can enhance the effects of the other essential oils. It can also impact your insulin levels and improve circulation and digestion. It can act as a gentle detoxifier in the body and stimulate the immune system. In aromatherapy, cinnamon essential oil is said to increase self-love and can improve your body image.

Bergamot

Although bergamot oil does not direct curb your appetite, it can effectively sooth your mind and relive stress. This can drastically improve your sense of well being and help you control food cravings. Since most people turn to food whenever they feel stressed, smelling bergamot oil can keep them from binging if they are not truly hungry.

Tangerine

This citrus essential oil can help you lose weight. Some people use it to tone their skin and reduce the appearance of cellulite and stretch marks. Tangerine oil is also said to be effective in regulating ones metabolism and can create the feeling of happiness. As a precaution, avoid direct sunlight right after applying the oil since it can increase light sensitivity. Tangerine essential oil is usually combined with other essential oils like lavender and bergamot.

Rose Geranium

Rose geranium is effective in lifting you mood. It also has properties which can reduce cellulite and can relive the symptoms of fluid retention. It is also effective in balancing your hormones. As an additional benefit, it has anti-fungal and anti-parasite agents.

Ocotea oil

Ocotea essential oil is extracted from a tree found in the Ecuador. Its flavor and aroma closely resembles cinnamon which is popular for its aromatic and medicinal properties. This is a rare type of essential oil which is found to help in controlling blood glucose level and lower cortisol levels. It can also help reduce your appetite. People who used this essential oil experienced an improvement in the blood sugar levels and had fewer food cravings.

Sandalwood oil

Just like bergamot oil, sandalwood essential oil can also help relieve stress related binging. It can improve your sense of well being and regain control over your habits. Sandalwood oil has long been used in different cultures to promote positive emotion and to help people overcome anxiety and depression.

Possible uses

You can use the essential oils to create your own blend and experiment to see what combination works for you.

- **Appetite balance**

2 drops tangerine oil

1 drop lavender oil

Combine the essential oils in a container then add it to your diffuser. You can also inhale from the bottle as often as desired.

- **Blood sugar control**

5 drops of ocotea oil

2 drops peppermint

1 oz jojoba oil

Massage the essential oils in your feet once or twice a day.

- **Cellulite control**

2 drops grapefruit

2 drops lavender oil

Mix the oils then use as massage oil and apply to your body daily.

- **Metabolism boosting**

2 drops cinnamon

2 drops ginger

1 drop peppermint

Add the essential oil in a bowl then combine it. Massage into your feet reflex points.

- **Sugar cravings**

2 drops ocotea oil

2 drops bergamot oil

4 drops peppermint oil

Combine in a bottle then inhale as needed.

- **Peppermint curb**

5 drops peppermint oil

Gently drop the essential oil in a handkerchief and inhale its scent before eating. You will automatically feel fuller and you will be able to control your appetite better.

- **Lemon coconut massage blend**

4 drops lemon oil

1 tsp virgin coconut oil

Pour the coconut oil in your palms and add the lemon oil. Massage all over your body paying close attention to your hips, belly and thighs.

- **Ocotea oil help**

Place few drops of ocotea oil under your tongue to help control your blood sugar. You can use this three times a day.

Sandalwood blend

5 drops sandalwood oil

5 drops jojoba oil

Combine the essential oils together then apply it directly into your feet.

- **Clary sage blend**

3 drops clary sage

3 drops jojoba oil

4 drops extra virgin coconut oil

Combine the oils then use topically. It is highly recommended that you apply it directly over your heart and along the length of your arms.

- **Lemongrass cholesterol control**

5 drops lemongrass oil

5 tsp honey

Mix the honey and essential oil in a small tea cup. Drink it straight then drink a glass of water. Lemon grass is known to lower cholesterol levels and can help minimize cravings.

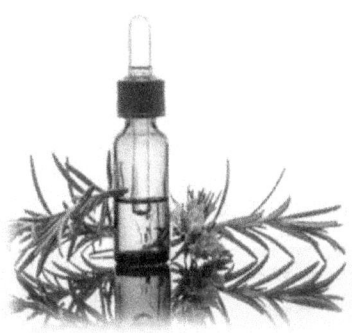

Chapter 8: Essential oil recipes for energy and happiness

Confidence boosting bergamot bath oil

3 drops bergamot oil

2 drops bay laurel oil

2 tsp jojoba oil

The essential oils can be directly added to your bath water but it cannot stay mixed in the water for a long time. There is also a possibility that it well settle in one area of your body so be sure to mix the bath water occassionally.

Orange and rosemary oil

4 drops rosemary oil

6 drops orange oil

2 tsp coconut oil

Mix the essential oil in a small container before applying to your body. You can also add it to your bath water. Make sure that the oil is well blended before you submerge your body into the water.

Grapefruit express

3 drops cypress oil

4 drops grapefruit oil

Add the essential oils in your diffuser and use as necessary. Store your aromatic blend in a dark glass bottle. Mix the oils together by rolling the bottle between your palms before using.

Energizing bergamot and jasmine

2 drops jasmine oil

8 drops bergamot oil

You may choose to add carrier oils like jojoba oil or coconut oil and use this blend as a massage oil or you can directly pour it in your diffuser and use as necessary.

Invigorating lemon peppermint air freshener

40 drops peppermint oil

40 drops lemon oil

20 drops Frankincense oil

1/5 oz high proof alcohol

Use a clean spray bottle with a fine mist setting. Avoid using bottles that have previously contained other products. Pour the essential oils into the bottle then roll at the palm of your hands to combine. Spray as necessary.

Fruity floral energizing air mist

20 drops rosemary

2 drops spearmint

4 drops peppermint

8 drops grapefruit

1.5 oz high proof alcohol

Combine the ingredients in a clean bottle. Be sure to spray away from furniture since the alcohol in this recipe can leave white spots in wood furnishings.

Pick me up massage oil

10 drops lime

2 drops rose oil

4 drops ylang ylang

7 drops bergamot oil

1 oz coconut oil

Mix the oils in a dark colored bottle. Shake well to combine before using as massage oil.

Bergamot and spearmint air freshener

15 drops spearmint oil

15 drops bergamot

Pour the oils in a spray bottle. Add distilled water or alcohol. You can try to reduce the oils and test it out first. Remember that different essential oils can have different aromatic strength. Also, it is wise to let it set for few hours before deciding to add more oil since essential oil aroma can change after it is sprayed into a room.

Grapefruit and ginger bath salts

3 drops grapefruit oil

2 drops ginger oil

½ cup Epsom salt

Pour the bath salt in a plate then gently add the essential oils. This recipe is good for one bath. You can double or triple the ingredients and store it in a glass bottle for future use.

Mystical energy diffuser blend

3 drops geranium oil

4 drops orange oil

4 drops Frankincense oil

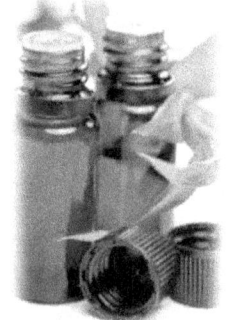

Gently drop the essential oils in a dark glass bottle then roll in your palms. Add the desired number of essential oil drops into your diffuser and use as instructed. You can also pour it in your handkerchief and smell the aroma directly from it.

Citrusy energizing blend

5 drops lemon or orange essential oil

3 drops ylang ylang

2 drops grapefruit oil

Combine the essential oil in your palms and use as massage oil. You can also add it to unscented body lotion and apply it as a cream over your body. Avoid applying this blend in the morning or before you go out since it contains citrus oils which can increase your photosensitivity.

Rose sandalwood bath oil

4 drops rose oil

8 drops sandalwood oil

2 tbsp jojoba oil

Combine the oils in a container then pour in your bath tub. Stir for few seconds before going in.

Celebratory essential blend

22 drops bergamot oil

10 drops cypress oil

5 drop ylang ylang oil

10 drops grapefruit oil

7 drops Frankincense

3 drops ginger oil

Combine the oil in a clean bottle glass and use as a diffuser. Bergamot has a light and sweet scent that can instantly lift your mood. Ylang ylang and cypress essential oil provides the blend with exotic aroma. However, the scent can be overpowering so try to use it sparingly.

Winter warming massage oil

4 oz natural base oil like olive or avocado oil

5 drops cypress essential oil

4 drops sandalwood essential oil

6 drops of orange essential oil

4 drops jasmine essential oil

4 drops rose oil

Add the ingredients in a dark bottle. Swirl the bottle after each essential oil is added. Once everything is thoroughly mixed, pour the base oil. Swirl for the last time. Apply to your skin as needed. This can help moisturize and revitalize your skin during cold nights.

Revitalizing winter bath salts

1 cup Epsom salt

6 drops bergamot essential oil

5 drops ginger oil

1 cup sea salt

5 drops rose oil

3 drops Frankincense oil

Mix the salt in a bowl. Gently mix in the essential oils and stir using a wooden spoon. When done, add the scented salts into your bath water. You can also use ¼ cup of this mixture for an energizing foot bath.

Chapter 9: Essential Oil Recipes for Your Home

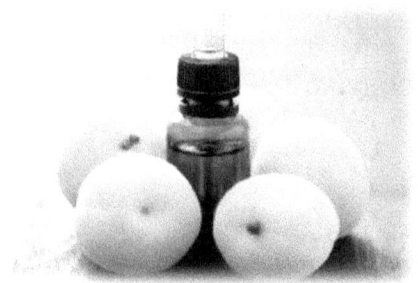

Carpet deodorizer

15 oz baking soda

10 drops orange or lemon essential oil

20 drops lavender oil

Place the baking soda in a bowl then gently pour the essential oils. Mix the oils together to reduce the risk of staining your carpet. This deodorizer can be stored in a glass container or plastic sifter. Shake the container before using. Sprinkle the mixture into your carpet. Leave it on your carpet for 20 minutes before vacuuming.

Dryer sheet recipe

5 drops lavender/ rose or chamomile oil

Scraps off white fabric

This dryer sheet can help make your laundry smell naturally fresh without having to spend money on expensive commercial dryer sheets. You will also avoid any synthetic chemical that it may contain. Drop the essential oils in the cotton fabric then place it in your dryer. Use as you normally would. Avoid using more than 5 drops of essential oil since they are flammable. Also, do not use colored fabric since it can stain you clothes.

Bed Linen recipes

Bed linen spray can keep your sheets smelling fresh between washes.

- **Relaxing spray**

8 drops mandarin oil

8 drops lavender oil

8 drops clary sage

20 drops Roman Chamomile oil

15 drops Bergamot oil

- **Citrus clean**

10 drops lemon oil

8 drops lavender oil

7 drop ginger oil

- **Sensual spray blend**

16 drops grapefruit

2 drops jasmine

13 drops sandalwood

4 drops rose oil

- **Exotic blend**

3 drops lime oil

4 drops ylang ylang

3 drops ginger oil

4 drops jasmine oil

2 drops rose oil

Choose one of the recipes above and pour the essential oils in a clean spray bottle with a mist system. Avoid using hair spray containers. Pour 1 to 2 ounces of distilled water or alcohol. Make sure to leave enough space in the bottle so that you can shake it before using. Spray into your bed linens and allow to sit for several minutes before hopping in. Be sure to use only light colored essential oils to make sure that it does not stain your linens. Do not spray directly into furniture.

Potpourri recipes

Potpourri is a mixture of flower, spices and essential oils. It literally means rotten pot. It is originally made from fermented layers of flowers and herbs which created a long lasting smell.

- **Basic rose potpourri**

3 cups rose petals

2 cups rosebuds

1 cup rose leaves

15 drops rose essential oil

2 cups lavender

2 tbsp powdered orris roots

Spread the fresh rose petals in a tray and place them in a warm and dry place. Spread them around every day until they are competently dry. Place the petals in a bowl. Add the orris root and stir to combine. Gently pour the essential oil and mix using your hands. Place in a paper bag and seal with clips. Shake the bag to ensure that the scent is evenly distributed. Store it away from direct sunlight.

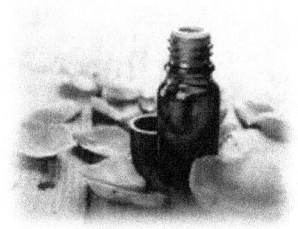

- **Citrus Zing**

1 oz lemon thyme

1 oz lemon verbena

1 oz lemon balm

2 drops lemon oil

½ oz marjoram

1 tbsp crushed lemon peel

2 drops orange blossom oil

2 tbsp orris root powder

¼ oz crumbled bay leaf

Mix all of the ingredients in a metal container then pour the oil. Stir to mix well. This recipe makes one cup. Place in your kitchen or laundry room. You can also add it in a diffuser lamp. Once it is heated, it will emit a stronger scent.

- **Holiday potpourri scent**

1 cup cinnamon sticks broken into pieces

1 cup dried orange peel

1 cup coriander

½ cup whole cloves

½ cup pine needles, fresh

½ cup orris root granules

5 drops of orange oil

1 cup all spice

1 cup bay leaves, broken into pieces

1 cup mint

½ cup star anise

½ cup rosemary leaves

10 drops cinnamon oil

Mix the cinnamon and orange essential oil in a small glass bowl. Set it aside while you combine the other ingredients in another glass bowl. Mix the ingredients using your hands. Store in a glass container and keep away from heat until you are ready to use. Place the mixture in the pan and add the water.

- **Soul soother**

2 oz rose petals

½ oz hibiscus flowers and lemon balm

1 tbsp crushed cinnamon sticks

2 tsp crushed cloves

3 tbsp carnation essential oil

1 oz chamomile flowers

8 crushed bay leaves

1 tbsp crushed vanilla pod

2 tsp crushed allspice

3 drops violet oil

Use rubber gloves and mix all of the ingredients together in a bowl except for the essential oils. Once the mixture is blended, add the oils gently and stir.

- **Pine and needles**

6 cups dried pine needles

2 cups dried orange peels

1 cup rose petals

4 tbsp orrisroot grains

2 cups white pine bark

1 cup dried rosehips

1 cup cinnamon sticks

15 drops pine essential oils

Place the orrisroot in a jar. Drop the pine essential oil then mix. Set aside and mix with the rest of the ingredients. Store it in an airtight container. Store it for six weeks. Make sure to stir it every week. To use, place into an open bowl. Remember that heat can enhance the scent.

- **Oriental jasmine**

2 oz rose petals, jasmine flowers and orange peel

¼ oz ginger root, crushed and broken into pieces

2 tsp crushed coriander seed

3 tbsp gum benzoin

1 oz sweet basil and sandalwood chips

2 tsp crushed anise seed

2 tsp cumin seed

6 drops jasmine essential oil

Place the ingredients in a bowl except for the oil. Stir it together to combine. Add the oil and mix again.

- **Spiced cones**

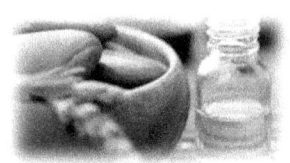

3 cups small pinecones

10 anise stars

½ cup allspice

½ cup orrisroot

10 drops or clove oil

1 cup white pine bark broken into pieces

1 cup broken cinnamon stick

½ cup cloves

¼ cup bay leaves

Pour the oil in the orrisroot. Gently mix then set it aside. Mix the ingredients together in a glass jar. Store it for six weeks. To stir, you can simply roll it back and forth. Do not remove the cover until ready to use. Place it in open containers around the house.

- **Country comfort**

1 oz of woodruff

3 crumble bay leaves

1 tbsp orris root

½ oz southernwood

2 tsp rosemary

Combine the ingredients in a bowl then transfer to a glass jar. Set aside for 6 weeks before using.

- **Pillow talk**

1 oz rose petals

1 oz lavender

2 tsp crushed cloves

½ oz lemon verbena

1 tbsp orris root

This potpourri recipe can induce sleep and help you relax at the same time. Combine the ingredients together in a bowl. Heat it to intensify the aroma.

- **Antibacterial herbs**

4 cups warm water

1/2 cup washing soda

20 drops thyme oil

Place the ingredients in a bowl then stir to combine the ingredients together. Pour in the container of your choice. Use it like regular disinfectant spray then wipe cloth.

- **Citrus dishwashing blend**

Liquid castile soap

10 drops sweet orange essential oil

20 drops lime essential oil

5 drops citrus seed extract

Dishwashing companies always use lemon scent in their products because of its natural antiseptic qualities. You can also create your own dishwashing blend without the harmful chemicals. Fill a squirt bottle with the soap. Add the essential oil and shake the bottle to combine. Add 1 tablespoon of the mixture into your dishwater.

- **Easy sink scrub**

¼ cup baking soda

¾ cup vinegar for rinsing

¼ cup baking soda

¾ cup vinegar

5 drops lemon oil

3 drops lavender oil

Mix the baking soda, washing soda and oils in a container. Stir well to combine then sprinkle into the skin. Let it stand for several minutes then scrub with hot water and vinegar.

- **Simple dishwasher powder**

3 cups washing soda

1 cup baking soda

5 drops lemon or orange oil

Combine the ingredients in a container. Add 2 tablespoon of the mixture into your dishwasher. You can easily double or triple the ingredients to make a larger bulk.

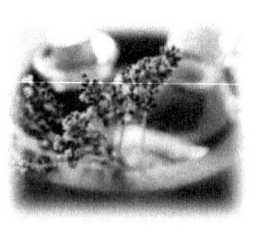

- **Oven stain removing formula**

½ cup salt

16 oz baking soda

¾ cup white vinegar

10 drops lemon grass essential oil

¼ cup washing soda

¼ cup water

10 drops thyme essential oil

This is a great stain remover for ovens. Pour the mixture into the oven then use a steel wood scrub to buff the surface.

- **Germs away toilet cleaner**

2 cups water

1 tbsp tea tree essential oil

¼ cup liquid castile soap

10 drops peppermint essential oil

This antibacterial cleaner is good for cleaning toilet surface. Combine the ingredients in a bottle then shake well. Spray on the surface before wiping with damp cloth.

- **Peppermint carpet cleaner**

10 drops peppermint oil

5 drops lemon oil

3 cups water

¾ cup liquid soap

Place the ingredients a bowl then stir to combine. Pour into your carpet and wash as needed.

Soy candles

Soy candles burn longer than your standard candles. It is also more eco friendly and is better for your health.

- **Spicy patchouli candle**

20 drops patchouli oil

15 drops sweet orange oil

15 drops cinnamon oil

- **Fresh mint soy candle**

20 drops spearmint oil

15 drops palmarosa oil

15 drops peppermint oil

- **Floral lavender candles**

25 drops lavender

13 drop rose geranium oil

10 drops rosewood oil

- **Woodsy candle scent**

30 drops rosewood oil

10 drops ylang ylang oil

12 drops cedar wood oil

- **Soft sensual candle recipe**

35 drops sandalwood oil

3 drops vetiver oil

12 ylang ylang oil

Make sure that your candle containers are clean. Place the wick at the center of the jar. Use two Popsicle sticks to hold it at the center. Heat the jar using a blow dryer. Pour water into the bottom of a pan and let it simmer. Pour the soy wax chips into the pan. Heat and stir continuously until the mixture is completely melted. Add the desired candle dye. Be sure to add a lot of dye if you want to achieve a deep color. Stir until the dye is completely mixed into the wax. Add the essential oil blends and stir to combine. Pour the wax into your chosen container. Do this slowly to prevent it from spilling and to minimize air pockets. Trim the wick as necessary.

Conclusion

Thank you again for downloading this book!

I hope this book was able to help you to understand essential oils and their many uses.

The next step is to continue experimenting with different essential oil blends and find your signature scent and cure.

Finally, if you enjoyed this book, please take the time to share your thoughts and post a review on Amazon. We do our best to reach out to readers and provide the best value we can. Your positive review will help us achieve that. It'd be greatly appreciated!

Thank you and good luck!

Check Out My Other Books

Coconut Oil for Easy Weight Loss: A Step by Step Guide for Using Virgin Coconut Oil for Quick and Easy Weight Loss

http://www.amazon.com/Coconut-Oil-Easy-Weight-Loss-ebook/dp/B00JG8H8DE

Superfoods that Kickstart Your Weight Loss Learn How to Use 30 Superfoods to Boost Weight Loss, Immunity and to Live a Healthier Lifestyle

Carrier Oils for Beginners: Discover the Characteristics and Beauty and Health Benefits of Carrier Oils For mixing Aromatherapy Essential Oils

http://www.amazon.com/Carrier-Oils-Beginners-Characteristics-Aromatherapy-ebook/dp/B00K88GI2S

Natural Homemade Cleaning Recipes For Beginners: Essential Oil Recipes For Household Cleaning, Laundry & Toxic Free Living

http://www.amazon.com/Natural-Homemade-Cleaning-Recipes-Beginners-ebook/dp/B00K87UBQI

The Best Secrets of Natural Remedies: The Ultimate Guide to Natural Remedies to Prevent and Cure Illnesses, Cold and Flu for Your Family

http://www.amazon.com/Best-Secrets-Natural-Remedies-Illnesses-ebook/dp/B00JNDCOCM

The Hypothyroidism Handbook:An Everyday Guide to Natural Solutions of living with Hypothyroidism including increased energy, lasting weight loss, and general well-being http://www.amazon.com/Hypothyroidism-Handbook-Solutions-including-increased-ebook/dp/B00JNIGIV0

The Hyperthyroidism Handbook: An Everyday Guide to Natural Solutions of Living with Hyperthyroidism including Weight Gain, Increased Energy and General Well-being

http://www.amazon.com/Hyperthyroidism-Handbook-Solutions-including-Hypothyroidism-ebook/dp/B00JOHU5SM

Essential Oils & Weight Loss for Beginners: Ultimate Guide to Losing Weight, Increasing Energy, Balancing Metabolism & Appetite Using Essential Oils & Aromatherapy

http://www.amazon.com/Essential-Oils-Weight-Loss-Beginners-ebook/dp/B00JOFOWP6

Top Essential Oil Recipes: A Recipe Guide Of Natural, Non-Toxic Aromatherapy & Essential Oils for Healing Common Ailments, Beauty, Stress & Anxiety

http://www.amazon.com/Top-Essential-Oil-Recipes-Aromatherapy-ebook/dp/B00JY434E2

Soap Making For Beginners: A Guide to Making Natural Homemade Soaps from Scratch, Includes Recipes and Step by Step Processes for Making Soaps

http://www.amazon.com/Soap-Making-Beginners-Homemade-Processes-ebook/dp/B00JYKH75I

Body Butters For Beginners: Proven Secrets To Making All Natural Body Butters For Rejuvenating And Hydrating Your Skin

http://www.amazon.com/Body-Butters-Beginners-Rejuvenating-Hydrating-ebook/dp/B00K6LVV6A

Apple Cider Vinegar For Beginners: Proven Secrets Using Apple Cider Vinegar For Health, Weight Loss, and Skin Care

http://www.amazon.com/Apple-Cider-Vinegar-Beginners-Aromatherapy-ebook/dp/B00K6YY6HI

Homemade Body Scrubs & Masks For Beginners: 50 Proven All Natural, Easy Recipes For Body & Facial Masks To Exfoliate Nourish, & Care For Your Skin

http://www.amazon.com/Homemade-Body-Scrubs-Masks-Beginners-ebook/dp/B00K79D4SY

Essential Oils Box Set #1: Essential Oils & Weight Loss For Beginners (Ultimate Guide to Losing Weight, Increasing Energy, Balancing Metabolism & Appetite Using Essential Oils & Aromatherapy) + Top Essential Oil Recipes (A Recipe Guide of Natural, Non-Toxic Aromatherapy & Essential Oils for Healing Common Ailments, Beauty, Stress & Anxiety)

http://www.amazon.com/Essential-Oils-Box-Set-Aromatherapy-ebook/dp/B00K7Q8HRK

Essential Oils Box Set #2: Essential Oils & Weight Loss For Beginners (Ultimate Guide to Losing Weight, Increasing Energy, Balancing Metabolism & Appetite Using Essential Oils & Aromatherapy) + Top Essential Oil Recipes (A Recipe Guide of Natural, Non-Toxic Aromatherapy & Essential Oils for Healing Common Ailments, Beauty, Stress & Anxiety)

http://www.amazon.com/Essential-Oils-Box-Set-Aromatherapy-ebook/dp/B00K7Q8HRK

Box Set#3: Coconut Oil for Easy Weight Loss(A Step by Step Guide for Using Virgin Coconut Oil for Quick and Easy Weight Loss) + Apple Cider Vinegar(Proven Secrets Using Apple Cider Vinegar for Health, Weight Loss, and Skin Care)

http://www.amazon.com/Box-Set-Beginners-Aromatherapy-Essential-ebook/dp/B00K9TEGUW

Box Set #4: Body butters For Beginners(Proven Secrets To Making All Natural Body Butters For Rejuvenating And Hydrating Your Skin) & Top Essential Oil Recipes: A Recipe Guide Of Natural, Non-Toxic Aromatherapy & Essential Oils for Healing Common Ailments, Beauty, Stress & Anxiety

http://www.amazon.com/Box-Set-Butters-Beginners-Essential-ebook/dp/B00KA02F4Y

Box Set #5: Soap Making For Beginners(A Guide to Making Natural Homemade Soaps from Scratch, Includes Recipes and Step by Step Processes for Making Soaps) + Homemade Body Scrubs & Masks For Beginners(50 Proven All Natural, Easy Recipes For Body Scrub & Facial Masks To Efoliate, Nourish, & Care For Your Skin)

http://www.amazon.com/Box-Set-Beginners-Homemade-Recipes-ebook/dp/B00K9U3I2I

Box Set #6: Body Butters for Beginners (Proven Secrets To Making All Natural Body Butters For Rejuvenating And Hydrating Your Skin) +Homemade Body Scrubs & Masks For Beginners(50 Proven All Natural, Easy Recipes For Body Scrub & Facial Masks To Exfoliate, Nourish, & Care For Your Skin)

http://www.amazon.com/Box-Set-Beginners-Exfoliating-Moisturizing-ebook/dp/B00K9U3Y4O

Box Set #7: Top Essential Oils(A Recipe Guide Of Natural, Non-Toxic Aromatherapy & Essential Oils For Healing, Common Ailments, Beauty, Stress & Anxiety) & The Best Secrets Of Natural Remedies (The Ultimate Guide to Natural Remedies to Prevent and Cure Illnesses, Cold and Flu for Your Family)

http://www.amazon.com/Box-Set-Essential-Recipes-Remedies-ebook/dp/B00K9WPMQG

Box Set #8: Natural Homemade Cleaning Recipes For Beginners (Essential Oil Recipes for Household Cleaning, Laundry & Toxic Free Living) + Top Essential Oils(A Recipe Guide Of Natural, Non-Toxic Aromatherapy & Essential Oils For Healing, Common Ailments, Beauty, Stress & Anxiety)

http://www.amazon.com/Box-Set-Beginners-Essential-Aromatherapy-ebook/dp/B00KAMNGBS

Box Set #9: Essential Oils & Weight Loss for Beginners (Ultimate Guide to Losing Weight, Increasing Energy, Balancing Metabolism & Appetite Using Essential Oils & Aromatherapy) + Carrier Oils for Beginners (Discover the Characteristics and Beauty and Health Benefits of Carrier Oils for Mixing Aromatherapy Essential Oils)

http://www.amazon.com/Box-Set-Essential-Beginners-Aromatherapy-ebook/dp/B00KAODL6Q

Box Set #10: The Hyperthyroidism Handbook (An Everyday Guide to Natural Solutions of Living with Hyperthyroidism including Weight Gain, Increased Energy and General Well-being) + The Hypothyroidism Handbook (Everyday Guide to Natural Solutions of Living With Hypothyroidism Including Increased Energy, Lasting Weight Loss, and General Well-Being)

http://www.amazon.com/Box-Set-10-Hyperthyroidism-Hypothyroidism-ebook/dp/B00KAKMSBY

Box Set #11: Carrier Oils For Beginners (Discover the Characteristics and Beauty and Health Benefits of Carrier Oils for Mixing Aromatherapy Essential Oils) + Essential Oils & Aromatherapy for Beginners (Secrets to Beauty,

Health and Weight Loss Using Proven Essential Oil and Aromatherapy Recipes

http://www.amazon.com/Box-Set-Beginners-Essential-Aromatherapy-ebook/dp/B00KAONEQ8

Box Set #12: Essential Oils & Weight Loss For Beginners: (Ultimate Guide to Losing Weight, Increasing Energy, Balancing Metabolism & Appetite Using Essential Oils & Aromatherapy) + Top Essential Oil Recipes (A Recipe Guide of Natural, Non-Toxic Aromatherapy & Essential Oils for Healing Common Ailments, Beauty, Stress & Anxiety) + Carrier Oils For Beginners (Discover the Characteristics & Beauty & Health Benefits of Carrier Oils for Mixing Aromatherapy Essential Oils) + Essential Oils & Aromatherapy For Beginners (Secrets to Beauty & weight Loss Using Proven Essential Oil & Aromatherapy Recipes) + Natural Homemade Cleaning Recipes For Beginners (Essential Oil Recipes for Household Cleaning, Laundry & Toxic Free Living)

http://www.amazon.com/Box-Set-12-Essential-Aromatherapy-ebook/dp/B00KCBCHE4

BOX SET #13: Superfoods That Kickstart Your Weight Loss (Learn How to Use 30 Superfoods to Boost Weight Loss, Immunity and to Live a Healthier Lifestyle) + Essential Oils & Aromatherapy for Beginners (Secrets to Beauty, Health and Weight Loss Using Proven Essential Oil and Aromatherapy Recipes) + Body Butters For Beginners (Proven Secrets To Making All Natural Body Butters For Rejuvenating And Hydrating Your Skin) + Soap Making For Beginners (A Guide to Making Natural Homemade Soaps from Scratch, Includes Recipes and Step by Step Processes for Making Soaps) + Homemade Body Scrubs For Beginners (50 Proven All Natural, Easy Recipes For Body Scrub & Facial Masks To Exfoliate, Nourish, & Care For Your Skin) http://www.amazon.com/Box-Set-Superfoods-Kickstart-Aromatherapy-ebook/dp/B00KC8G6DK/

Box Set #14: Essential Oils & Weight Loss for Beginners (Ultimate Guide to Losing Weight, Increasing Energy, Balancing Metabolism & Appetite Using Essential Oils & Aromatherapy) + Apple Cider Vinegar for Beginners (Proven Secrets Using Apple Cider Vinegar for Health, Weight Loss, and Skin Care) + Body Butters For Beginners (Proven Secrets To Making All Natural Body Butters For Rejuvenating And Hydrating Your Skin)
+ Homemade Body Scrubs & Masks for Beginners (50 Proven All Natural, Easy Recipes for Body Scrub & Facial Masks to Exfoliate, Nourish, & Care for Your Skin) + Coconut Oil for Easy Weight Loss (A Step by Step Guide for Using Virgin Coconut Oil for Quick and Easy Weight Loss)

http://www.amazon.com/Box-Set-Essential-Beginners-Aromatherapy-ebook/dp/B00KEDO68U

If the links do not work, for whatever reason, you can simply search for these titles on the Amazon website to find them.

www.ingramcontent.com/pod-product-compliance
Lightning Source LLC
Chambersburg PA
CBHW060154290526
45789CB00003B/1039